Paleo Diet For Beginners Quickstart Guide

How To Start The Paleo Diet With These Easy Paleo Diet Recipes For Weight Loss

Sarah Joy

Table of Contents

Introduction

I want to thank you and congratulate you for buying the book, *"Paleo Diet For Beginners Quickstart Guide - How To Start The Paleo Diet With These Easy Paleo Diet Recipes For Weight Loss"*.

How do you start on a Paleo diet? This is the question that most people have. The greatest challenge is not usually the zeal and the motivation to start on the paleo diet but rather how to get easy and delicious recipes to get started on the Paleo Diet. We have been made to believe that you have not eaten any meal unless you have some grains. However, do you know that some of these grains are the reason for all the problems that we are currently facing like obesity.

If you want to lose weight and keep off the weight, the trick is to eat like the caveman did. Did the caveman grow grains? Did they drink milk? No, the caveman was busy hunting and gathering his food. Adapting the caveman diet will not only help you live a healthy and fulfilling life knowing that you are consuming real food but you will also be in a position to lose weight. Who does not want to have that nice slim figure?

This book has amazing recipes to get you started on your journey to eating like the caveman; I have compiled breakfast, lunch, dinner and dessert recipes. With this book, be rest assured that you will have no problem starting the Paleo diet as the recipes are simple, easy to make and delicious. No need to skip meals or just take cabbage soup to lose weight; you can still lose weight and eat amazing meals. Losing weight has never been this easy, fun and amazing.

Thanks again for downloading this book, I hope you enjoy it!

The Paleo Diet: Eating Like The Caveman

Did you know that the invention of agriculture and domestication of animals only took place about 10,000 years ago? What then did man eat? The Paleolithic man ate wild fruits, wild vegetables and game meat. What then does the current man eat? Our diet is high in refined carbohydrates and sugars and low in vegetables and fruits. When you compare the Paleolithic man and the current man, you can clearly tell the difference. The caveman was athletic, strong, muscular and agile while the current man is overweight, lacks energy and stressed. What then could be the problem? Even with the invention of agriculture and the beginning of man to grow grains to make provision of food easier, our body was not used to the consumption of grains. Actually, our bodies have not adapted to consumption of some of these grains that are high in gluten for instance which has negative effects like causing inflammation. Domestication of animals and consumption of milk also has its own shares of problems with some people being lactose sensitive.

The only way that you can lose weight and keep the weight off is to eat what works with our bodies. The paleo diet has a simple approach to eating; it is as simple as if the caveman didn't eat it, you shouldn't either. The greatest problem for many people who want to start on the Paleo diet is what to eat and what to avoid. We will thus look at the different things you can eat as well as what you can avoid when on a Paleo diet.

What to Avoid

Grains: This includes pastas, wheat, rye, barley, spelt and breads.

Legumes: This includes lentils, beans and all legumes.

Sugar and High Fructose Corn Syrup: This includes foods high in sugar like candy, pastries, tables sugar, soft drinks and ice cream.

Trans Fats: These are found in margarine and most processed foods that use margarine. Trans fats may also be referred to as "partially hydrogenate or "hydrogenated". You should avoid foods with these words.

Vegetable Oils: This includes corn oil, sunflower oil, grapeseed oil, safflower oil and many others.

Dairy: Avoid most dairy. This is a grey area for most people especially since dairy products are high in calcium. If you have to take dairy products, ensure that they are from grass-fed animals.

Artificial Sweeteners and Alcohol

What You can Eat

Now that you know what foods you need to avoid, let us look at what you can eat.

*Lean Meats like beef, chicken turkey, pork, lamb and game meat

*Vegetables such as kale, peppers, carrots, onions, cauliflower, cabbage, broccoli, spinach, potatoes, yams, turnips and sweet potatoes

*Fruits like bananas, oranges, apples, avocadoes, pears, berries, pineapples, papaya

*Seafood and Fish like haddock, shrimp, trout, shrimp and salmon

*Nuts and seeds like walnuts, macadamia nuts, walnuts, hazelnuts, pumpkin and sunflower seeds

*Natural fats and oils such as coconut oil, avocado oil, olive oil and lard

*You can eat as much spices as you want. However, ensure that they are natural; no additives.

*You can also eat eggs although ensure that you use pastured eggs.

We now know what to eat and avoid so let's start cooking. We will look at breakfast, lunch, dinner and dessert recipes to get you started on your Paleo diet.

1. It still feels so unreal that my best friend, my grandfathe
   I know, spent days tanning with me and teaching me to
   everyone laughing until the end. He is truly the greatest
   grandpa

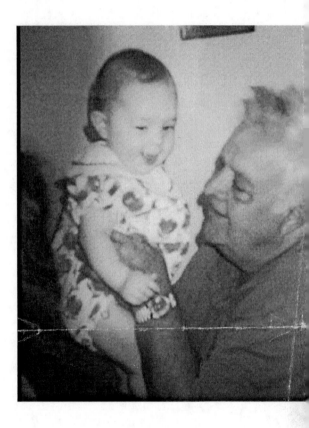

r, the man who helped raised me and taught me most of what
bay gin rummy, took me on field trips and most of all kept
man to ever live, fly high my angel I love you so much

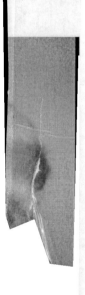

Horseradish Scrambled Eggs (225 Calories Per Serving)

Makes 2 Servings

Ingredients

- 4 slices of raw bacon
- 6 eggs
- 1 teaspoon of horseradish

Directions

1. Put the skillet over medium heat. Place the bacon into the skillet. Fry until crisp and once cooked, drain and crumble. Whisk all the eggs along with the horseradish.

2. Reserve one tablespoon of the grease to cook the eggs. Put the eggs into the skillet and cook until almost set. Add the bits of bacon and stir the mixture. Cook for around 3 minutes then serve.

Menemen (388 calories per serving)

Makes 2 Servings

Ingredients

- ¼ diced red onion.
- 1 medium tomato, ¼ inch diced
- 1 tablespoon olive oil
- 1 garlic clove, crushed
- ¼ teaspoon ground cumin
- ¼ teaspoon black pepper

- ¼ teaspoon turmeric
- ¼ teaspoon red pepper flakes
- 3 eggs
- ¼ teaspoon of salt
- 1 tablespoon minced fresh parsley

Directions

1. Sauté the onion, pepper, and tomato in olive oil in a heavy skillet over medium-low heat, Crush the garlic and put into the skillet then stir. Continue cooking while stirring often. While vegetables are cooking, put eggs in a bowl and whisk. When the vegetables are almost cooked, pour in eggs and cook until they are set. Scoop onto a plate and garnish with parsley then serve.

Cinnamon-Honey Paleonola (33 calories per serving)

Makes 16 Servings

Ingredients

- 2 cups of shredded coconut meat
- 1 cup flaxseed meal
- ½ cup of water
- 1 teaspoon ground cinnamon
- ½ cup coconut oil
- ½ cup chopped walnuts
- ½ cup honey
- ¼ cup of sesame seeds (optional)
- ½ teaspoon salt
- 2 cups of chopped pecans
- ½ cup sliced almonds

- ½ cup sunflower seeds
- ½ cup shelled pumpkin seeds

Directions

1. Preheat oven to 250 degrees F. Combine coconut, flaxseed, cinnamon, sesame seeds and salt. Stir to distribute them evenly. Pour the oil, honey and water over the dry ingredients. Stir to mix until everything is evenly damp. Put the mixture into an 11 x 13 inch roasting foil, press it into an even layer at the bottom of the pan and put in the oven. Set the timer for one hour.

2. After one hour, remove the pan from the oven. Use the edge of a spatula to cut the whole thing into 1-inch squares and then scoop up the chunks and stir them around in the pan. Cut into smaller pieces, stir in the nuts and seeds, place the pan back in the oven and set timer for 20 minutes. Repeat for two or three times, until the nuts and seeds are roasted. Remove from oven, let cool it cool, store in an airtight container and serve with coconut milk.

Baked Eggs with Bacon and Spinach (284 calories per servings)

Makes 2 Servings

Ingredients

- 4 large eggs
- 1 5-ounce bag baby spinach
- 4 tablespoons heavy whipping cream
- 6 slices of applewood-smoked bacon

8

Directions

1. Preheat oven to 400°F. Cook bacon in a large skillet over medium heat until crisp. Move to paper towels and drain the grease. Add spinach to the pan and sprinkle with pepper. Toss over medium heat for 1 minute and transfer to strainer set over bowl to drain. Take ramekins and brush with dripping. Crumble bacon.

2. Share the spinach among ramekins and then sprinkle bacon over ensuring to divide equally. Shape and create a well at the center with a spoon. Crack 1 egg into well in each ramekin ensuring to keep the yolk intact. Put 1 tablespoon cream over each egg then sprinkle with salt and pepper and bake eggs until whites are just set but yolks are still moist then serve.

Chorizo and Scrambled Egg Breakfast Tacos (412 calories per serving)

Makes 4 Servings

Ingredients

- 4 large eggs
- 4 green onions, sliced
- 1 cup of grated cheddar cheese (grass-fed)
- 4 flaxseed tortillas
- Hot sauce or salsa (optional)
- 7 ounces fresh chorizo sausage
- 4 tablespoons of chopped fresh cilantro, divided
- Sour cream (optional)

Directions

1. Brush a large nonstick pan using olive oil then char the tortillas directly on electric burner until they are blackened in spots while turning using tongs then arrange the tortillas in a single layer in the pan and spread each tortilla with ¼ cup of grated cheese and put aside. Whisk 2 tablespoons cilantro and eggs in a medium bowl then season with pepper and salt. Cook the sausage in a medium non-stick pan over medium heat until cooked, break the bacon using the back of the spoon and add green onions and sauté. Add egg mixture and stir then cook until almost set then remove egg mixture from heat.

2. Cook the tortillas in skillet over high heat until crisp on bottom. Divide the egg mixture among the tortillas and then sprinkle with the remaining cilantro, wrap each tortilla in half and serve.

Baked Eggs in Bacon Rings (108 calories per serving)

Makes 2 Servings

Ingredients

- 4 eggs
- Melted bacon fat for brushing tins
- 1 tomato, cut into 4 (½ inch) slices
- 6 strips of nitrate or nitrite free bacon
- ½ teaspoon freshly ground black pepper
- 1/3 cup onions, chopped
- 3-4 white button mushrooms, chopped

Directions

1. Preheat oven to 325°F. Put bacon in a skillet over medium heat and sauté for 3 minutes. Discard the bacon fat except a little at the bottom of the skillet. Brush 4 cups in a muffin tin with bacon fat. Put chopped onions and mushrooms in the bacon drippings in the hot skillet and cook until softened.

2. Put a slice of tomato in the bottom of each cup. Take ½ strips of bacon and circle the inside of the cups. Put an egg into each muffin cup, season with pepper and then add the sautéed onions and mushrooms over the egg and bake for 20 minutes. Loosen the edges of the eggs with spatula and transfer the eggs to plates then serve.

Sausage and Zucchini Breakfast Casserole (197 calories per serving)

Makes 4 servings

Ingredients

- 1 pound ground breakfast sausage
- 4 large white button mushrooms, halved
- 6 large eggs, beaten
- 2 tablespoons almond flour
- ½ teaspoon fresh thyme leaves (optional)
- 1-1/4 pound zucchini, trimmed
- ½ teaspoon granulated garlic
- 1 large yellow onion, peeled and quartered
- 1 teaspoon sea salt
- ¼ teaspoon cayenne (optional)

Directions

1. Preheat oven to 400 degrees F. Place a grater blade on a medium food processor and grate the zucchini, onion and mushrooms. Put the vegetable mixture into the bottom of a 9x9 baking dish and pat down lightly to form an even surface. Crumble the raw sausage on top of the vegetables and spread fresh thyme with almond flour.

2. In a medium mixing bowl, mix granulated garlic, eggs, sea salt, and cayenne and whisk until eggs are a pale yellow. Pour egg mixture evenly over vegetable and sausage and let it sink to the bottom of the pan.

3. Place in oven and bake for 45 to 55 minutes. Ignore the water from the vegetables. Let it cool for 15 minutes and slice into 4 servings.

Paleo Lunch Recipes

Standard Egg Salad (374 calories per serving)

Makes 4 Servings

Ingredients

- 2 large celery ribs, diced
- ½ green bell pepper, diced
- 4 scallions sliced thinly
- 2 tablespoons minced fresh parsley
- 6 hard boiled eggs, peeled, and chopped
- 1 tablespoon brown mustard Salt
- 6 tablespoons Mayonnaise
- Black pepper to taste

Directions

1. Chop the vegetables and combine with the eggs in a mixing bowl.

2. Stir together the mustard and the mayonnaise. Add the mixture to the salad and stir then add in salt and pepper to taste then serve.

Ceviche (221 calories per serving)

Makes 8 Servings

Ingredients

- 1 habanero chile or jalapeno
- 2 pounds fish fillets, cubed

- 8 garlic cloves
- 10 limes
- 1 tablespoon minced fresh cilantro
- Salt and pepper to taste
- 1 small red onion sliced
- 16 large romaine lettuce leaves
- 2 tomatoes, diced
- 2 avocados diced
- Hot sauce

Directions

1. Squeeze limes into a food processor then add cilantro and garlic into the processor and process a few times until well minced and then pour this mixture over the fish, slice onion and then add on the fish. Chill overnight to allow the fish to marinate. Stir once or twice and drain off most of the limejuice, add salt and pepper to taste then serve.

Chicken Salad (465 calories per serving)

Makes 3 Servings

Ingredients

- 1 cup diced cooked chicken
- 1 artichoke heart
- ⅓ cup of lemon-balsamic mayonnaise
- ½ cup diced red bell pepper
- 2 scallions
- 1 tablespoon minced fresh parsley

Directions

1. Put everything in a mixing bowl. Add the mayonnaise into the ingredients and coat.

Making Mayonnaise:

Put 2 egg yolks, 1 tablespoon lemon juice, 1 tablespoon vinegar, and ½ garlic clove into the bottom of a clean glass jar then add ¼-cup extra-virgin olive oil then dip a stick blender into the mixture then blend the mixture until smooth. Keeping the blender on, add in ⅔ cup of light-flavored olive oil into the mixture and process until you have a thick consistency and the oil starts paddling on the surface.

Chicken-Avocado Soup (277 calories per serving)

Makes 4 Servings

Ingredients

- 1 pound boneless chicken breast
- 6 cups chicken broth
- 1 teaspoon Sriracha
- 1 avocado
- 4 scallions
- 1 crushed clove garlic
- Salt and black pepper

Directions

1. Put broth into saucepan and place over medium-high heat then stir in Sriracha. Cut chicken into bite-size pieces, dice the avocado and slice the scallions. Separate

white and crisp green parts then stir in chicken and white part of scallions. Add in the crushed garlic and bring back to a simmer, reduce heat to low and simmer for 10 minutes then add salt and pepper to taste. Pour into bowls, separate avocado and sliced green scallion shoots among bowls then serve.

Ginger Tuna Ceviche (365 Calories Per Serving)

Makes 3 Servings

Ingredients

- 1 pound fresh tuna
- 1 loose handful fresh parsley leaves
- Freshly ground black pepper
- 2-inch piece of ginger
- 1 small mild chili, finely diced
- 1 handful of fresh finely chopped cilantro leaves
- 1 lime, juiced
- Olive oil

Directions

1. Grate ginger finely. Using small holes grater squeeze firmly, catching the juice in a bowl below.

2. Put the chili, finely chopped herbs and tuna into a mixing bowl. Stir the limejuice into the ginger juice and pour the juice over the other ingredients then mix well.

3. Let it sit for 30 minutes. Pour some olive oil into the fish and sprinkle with black pepper then serve.

Paleo Lamb With Rosemary (292 Calories Per Serving)

Makes 4 Servings

Ingredients

- 1 cup of sulphite-free red wine
- 1 pound of lamb ribs or steaks
- ¼ cup of balsamic vinegar
- 1 tablespoon of fresh cracked pepper
- 3 tablespoons of extra virgin olive oil
- 2 fresh organic sprigs of rosemary with leaves removed from stems

Directions

1. Put lamb in a 2-3 inch deep dish. Mix all other ingredients well. Pour over lamb ensuring that you coat the lamb. Cover and refrigerate for 1-2 days.

2. Barbeque lightly and turn to low heat then put lamb on grill and cook for 10-12 minutes each side, or until meat is cooked as desired.

3. Pour the remaining marinade over meat while cooking. Serve with fresh cantaloupe with a green salad and some steamed artichokes.

Persian-Inspired Dried Lime Chicken (306 Calories Per Serving)

Makes 4 Servings

Ingredients

- 2 pounds bone-in chicken pieces
- Slices of 2 dried limes
- 1 onion, finely diced
- ¾ cup fresh herbs (mixture of parsley, cilantro, and mint)
- 3 pressed cloves garlic
- 1 bell pepper
- 2 teaspoons turmeric
- 2 teaspoons cumin
- 2 teaspoons coriander powder
- 1 lemon, juiced
- Olive oil
- 2 teaspoons mild paprika
- Freshly ground black pepper

Directions

1. Break the dried limes into pieces and put in a bowl. Add a cup of boiling water and let settle for 15 minutes. Prepare the remaining ingredients.

2. Arrange onion, garlic, and bell pepper and set aside then prepare the herbs and spices. Chop the limes into small pieces. Mix the lime pieces and their soaking water with the garlic, onion, bell pepper, spices, herbs, lemon juice, and another ¾-cup water then stir well. Add the chicken pieces and sprinkle black pepper. Mix well and place the mixture in a baking dish.

18

3. Bake at 350°F for 1 hour. Stir the mixture every 20 minutes. The dish should remain very moist. Otherwise, add water and stir. Take out the chicken golden brown and tender then serve

Chicken Breasts With Portobello Mushrooms (350 Calories Per Serving)

Makes 4 Servings

Ingredients

- 4 free range organic chicken breast fillets, thoroughly rinsed
- 1 cup organic marsala wine
- 2 cups of organic portobello mushrooms, sliced and rinsed
- 2 tablespoons red wine vinegar
- 4 tablespoons of extra virgin olive oil
- 1 clove garlic
- 2 sprigs fresh rosemary
- 1 small sweet onion, thinly sliced
- Freshly cracked pepper to taste

Directions

1. Preheat oven to 375°F. Put chicken breasts in baking dish and cover with mushrooms. Mix wine, red wine vinegar, rosemary and 3 tablespoons extra virgin oil in a bowl then sauté garlic and onion with 1 tablespoon of the remaining olive oil in shallow pan, spread garlic and onions over the chicken and mushrooms and empty the liquid mixture over chicken and ensure that the

chicken is coated well with the mixture. Bake for 45 minutes and then serve hot.

Paleo Dinner Recipes

Gingery Broccoli Beef (331.1 Calories Per Serving)

Makes 4 servings

Ingredients

- 2 teaspoons black pepper
- 2 cloves of garlic, minced
- 2 cups carrots, thinly sliced
- 2 teaspoons freshly grated ginger
- 1 tablespoon Flax meal
- 2 tablespoons of coconut oil (separated)
- 1 green onion, thinly sliced
- ½ low sodium chicken broth
- 1 pound petite sirloin steak, sliced
- 2 broccoli, cut into florets
- ½ teaspoon of red pepper flakes
- Lemon juice
- ¼ teaspoon of sea salt

Directions

1. Heat 1 tablespoon coconut oil and garlic in a pan over medium high heat. Add sirloin and sea salt and sauté then remove the sirloin steak from pan and set aside. Drain juice from pan.

2. Mix lemon juice, ginger, black pepper, flax meal, and red pepper with broth in a separate bowl. Add broccoli and carrots to pan then pour the liquid ingredients and toss to coat.

3. Simmer until broccoli is tender. Return your beef back

to the pan. Add green onions and let it simmer until beef has been re-warmed then serve.

Beef And Veg Chili (205.5 Calories per serving)

Makes 3 servings

Ingredients

- 0.3 pounds lean minced beef
- 0.8 pounds tomatoes
- ½ dried chili
- 1 tablespoon Worcestershire sauce
- 50g pepper
- 200g tin red kidney beans
- 1 medium onion
- 60g mushrooms
- Cumin coriander and chili powder
- 90g celery

Directions

1. Fry the minced beef, ensuring to pour off any excess fat. Add 2 chopped cloves of garlic then fry a little and add the chopped onions. Add the rest of the chopped vegetables and cook a little longer then add half-dried chopped chili with the fine seeds removed.

2. Add half teaspoon each of cumin and coriander, hot chili powder along with a tablespoon of Worcestershire sauce.

3. Add the tin of chopped tomatoes and the tin of red kidney beans then season with salt if needed and black

pepper. Cook for 1 hour and serve hot.

Zucchini And Ground Beef (353.4 Calories Per Serving)

Makes 4 servings

Ingredients

- 2 cups of water
- 1 pound ground beef
- 2 large zucchini
- ½ teaspoon of curry
- 1 can of no-salt tomato sauce

Directions

1. Brown the ground beef and remove the excess fat. Cut the zucchini into chunks and boil until soft. Mix this with meat and add water, spices and the can of tomato sauce.

2. Let it boil and reduce the heat. Let it sit for a few minutes to take in the spices then serve.

Baked Chicken Fajitas (304.1 Calories Per Serving)

Makes 8 servings

Ingredients

- 16 ounce frozen boneless chicken breasts
- 2 teaspoons chili

- 2 teaspoons cumin
- Raw sliced green peppers
- 2 tablespoons canola oil
- 1 can diced sweet onion
- 1 cup raw onions
- 8 flaxseed tortillas

Directions

1. Cut chicken into strips. Cut onion and both peppers into strips.

2. Combine all other ingredients and stir. Add chicken, peppers and onions and toss to coat then add the chicken mixture to a sprayed 13x9" casserole dish and bake until the chicken is cooked through and onions are done, about 20-25 minutes. Serve on flaxseed tortilla shells.

Sesame Chicken (643.9 Calories Per Serving)

Makes 2 Servings

Ingredients

- 4 tablespoons soy sauce, low sodium
- 1 tablespoon olive oil
- 2 chicken breasts, no skin
- 1 tablespoon of sesame seeds
- 2 tablespoons of honey
- 2 cups broccoli, cooked

Directions

1. Mix soy sauce, honey and sesame seeds in a small bowl. Steam broccoli, set aside to drain well, cube chicken into 1.5 pieces and fry in olive oil. Add broccoli to pan with chicken, then pour over sauce. Stir and serve with some potatoes.

Honey Garlic Pork Chops (204.3 Calories Per Serving)

Makes 6 Servings

Ingredients

- 6 cloves garlic, minced
- 6 (4 pound) boneless pork loin chops
- 3 tablespoons of soy sauce
- 1/3 cup of honey, divided

Directions

1. Whisk together garlic, honey and soy sauce in a shallow dish. Coat chops in the mixture, reserve any remaining honey mixture to use for basting then place the chops on greased grill over medium high heat and close the lid. Cook while basting 2 times and serve hot.

Buffalo Turkey Burgers (153.3 Calories per serving)

Makes 5 servings

Ingredients

- ¼ cup garlic
- 2/3 cup grated carrots
- 16-ounce ground turkey (93% lean)
- 1 teaspoon Tabasco sauce

Directions

- Mix all ingredients together. Form five patties. Make into a patty then grill for four minutes each side on an indoor grill on medium heat and serve.

Paleo Dessert Recipes

Dark Chocolate Fudge Pops (145 Calories Per Serving)

Makes 5 Servings

Ingredients

- 1 ¼ cups coconut milk
- 2 egg yolks
- ½ cup honey
- Dash of sea salt
- 1 ½ teaspoons gelatin (unflavored)
- 1 teaspoon vanilla extract
- 2 ounces unsweetened chocolate, chopped roughly

Directions

1. Place the gelatin in a small bowl with vanilla extract to soften it. Warm the coconut milk over medium-high heat for 6-7 minutes (should not boil).

2. Whisk the egg yolks, salt and honey in a small bowl. Pour the hot coconut milk slowly into the egg mixture. Whisk continuously to temper the eggs.

3. Pour the entire liquid mixture back into the pan, and continue cooking over medium-high heat for 6-8 minutes. Stir constantly and ensure that it does not boil. The mixture should be thick enough to coat the back of a spoon.

4. Pour the softened vanilla and gelatin into the pan. Whisk until the gelatin has dissolved completely. Remove from the heat and pour the mixture into a glass

bowl.

5. Stir in the chopped chocolate. Let the pudding cool for around 20 minutes at room temperature.

6. Pour the pudding into Popsicle molds and freeze until solid, then serve.

Paleo Chocolate Lasagna (240.3 Calories Per Serving)

Makes 2 Servings

Ingredients

- ½ cup grass-fed butter
- ½ cup coconut oil, plus more for greasing the pan
- 1 & 1/3 cups coconut palm sugar
- 1 teaspoon vanilla
- ½ teaspoon sea salt
- 1 teaspoon baking soda
- 2 organic pastured eggs
- ½ cup creamy almond butter
- ½ cup coconut flour
- ¾ cup unsweetened cocoa powder
- 1/2 cup canned coconut milk, full-fat
- ½ teaspoon baking powder
- 2 teaspoons apple cider vinegar
- 1 cup shredded zucchini (with peel)
- 1 cup Chocolate Chips

Directions

1. Preheat the oven to 350°F. Lightly grease a 9 x 13 glass pan with butter or coconut oil. In a large mixing bowl, put butter, vanilla, coconut oil, coconut palm sugar, baking powder, salt, and baking soda then beat in the eggs and mix thoroughly. Stir in the coconut milk, almond butter, coconut flour, and apple cider vinegar. Add in the cocoa, and mix until smooth. Fold in the zucchini and a cup of chocolate chips. You can then spoon the batter into the greased 9 x 13 glass pan, bake for 30-35 minutes or until a toothpick comes out clean. Prepare the center chocolate pudding layer and the top whipped cream frosting layer as you let the cake cool.

Middle Layer: Paleo Chocolate Pudding

Ingredients

- 6 medjool dates
- ¾ cup unsweetened cocoa powder
- 4 ripe avocados
- ½ cup pure maple syrup
- 2 teaspoons vanilla extract
- 4 tablespoons of unsweetened vanilla almond milk
- Dash of sea salt
- Dash of cinnamon

Directions

1. Place the dates in a bowl of warm water in order to soften them. Cut avocados in half, remove the pits and scoop the avocados out with a spoon into a food

processor; the avocados should be soft and ripe. Remove the pits from the dates and tear them in half. Add the other ingredients into the food processor and puree until you achieve a pudding like consistency then transfer from the food processor into a bowl. Place in the fridge.

Paleo Whipped Cream Frosting: Top Layer

Ingredients

- ¼ cup pure maple syrup
- ¼ cup unsweetened vanilla almond milk
- ½ cup canned coconut milk, full fat
- 2 tablespoons coconut oil (melted)
- ¼ cup coconut flour
- 1 cup organic palm shortening
- 1 tablespoon raw honey
- 2 teaspoons vanilla
- 1 tablespoon arrowroot powder
- Pinch of sea salt
- Pinch of cinnamon
- 1 cup Chocolate Chips

Directions

1. Mix all ingredients except chocolate chips in a food processor and process until well combined. Transfer whipped cream into a bowl, place in the fridge and let the cake completely cool. Take the Paleo Chocolate Pudding and spread a thick layer on top of the cake like frosting. Take the Whipped Cream Frosting and spread on top of Paleo Chocolate Pudding layer. Use fingers,

spatula and knives to spread on the top without mixing the chocolate pudding layer into it. Sprinkle Chocolate Chips all across the top to garnish the Lasagna. Use melted chocolate for decorations.

Almond Butter Banana Cookies (154 Calories Per Serving)

Makes 16 Servings

Ingredients

- 3 medjool dates, pits removed
- 2 ripe bananas
- ¼ teaspoon ground cloves
- ½ cup of crushed pecans
- ½ cup of almond butter
- 1 egg
- ½ teaspoon vanilla extract
- ½ teaspoon nutmeg
- ½ teaspoon baking soda

Directions

1. Preheat oven to 350 Degrees Fahrenheit. Put dates in the food processor and pulse until finely chopped. Add bananas, butter, almond, egg, and vanilla extract and process until a smooth batter with small chunks is obtained. Add in cloves, baking soda, nutmeg and crushed pecans. Mix thoroughly to obtain an even distribution of all ingredients. Take a medium sized cookie scoop. Take one scoop of the batter onto a baking sheet lined with parchment paper. Ensure you

leave enough space for the mixture to spread out.

2. Bake until golden brown on the bottom. Remove from the oven and allow to cool.

Mint Chip Ice Cream (160 Calories Per Serving)

Makes Servings 4

Ingredients

- 2 cups of cold almond milk
- 1 can of full fat coconut milk
- ½ cup of raw honey
- ¾ teaspoon peppermint extract
- 1 tablespoon coconut oil (melted)
- 1/3 cup diced avocado
- ½ cup of chopped dark chocolate

Directions

1. Place the coconut milk and mint leaves in a saucepan over medium-high heat for 10 minutes. Place the mint, honey and warm coconut milk in a medium-sized bowl. Mix until all the honey has dissolved completely. Stir in the peppermint extract and almond milk. Cover and put in the fridge for 4 hours. Pour the resultant mixture into a blender, add the coconut oil, avocado, and coloring if desired and blend until smooth. Place this mixture in an ice cream maker and follow the manufacturer's instructions to make ice cream. Immediately the mixture has achieved a soft serve consistency, add in the chocolate by hand. Spoon the ice

cream into an airtight container and freeze for about 2 hours or until firm. Serve immediately, or you can defrost in the fridge for one hour before serving.

Raw Dark Chocolate Blackberry Cheesecake (494 Calories Per Serving)

Makes 6 Servings

Ingredients

For the crust

- 10 medjool dates
- 2 cups raw almonds
- 8 tablespoons maple syrup
- ½ teaspoon sea salt
- 8 tablespoons cacao powder

For the filling

- 1 cup light coconut milk
- ½ cup coconut oil
- 2 cups raw cashews
- 2 teaspoons vanilla extract
- ½ cup maple syrup
- 8 tablespoons cacao powder

For the Blackberry sauce

- 12 ounces of fresh blackberry
- 6 tablespoons maple syrup
- ½ cup filtered water

Directions

1. Process all the crust ingredients in a food processor. Keep the nuts chunky. Test the crust by spooning out a small amount of the mixture. Make sure the ingredients hold together.

2. Scoop out crust mixture in a 9" cheesecake pan. Firmly press the mixture. Make sure the edges are well packed and the base is even.

3. For the filling, add maple syrup, soaked cashews, melted coconut oil, coconut milk, cacao powder and vanilla extract into the food processor and process on high until very smooth. Pour mixture on top of the crust and smooth evenly with a spatula.

4. Place cheesecake in the freezer until it becomes solid. Place saucepan under medium heat, add water, 6 tablespoons of maple syrup, and 6 ounces of blackberries and bring to a boil. Let I boil for about 12 minutes stirring constantly. Remove from heat and immediately add remaining 6 ounces of blackberries then stir and mix well and let cool before serving.

Paleo Apple Pie Cupcakes With Cinnamon Frosting (260calories Per Serving)

Makes 12 Servings

Ingredients

- 5 Eggs
- 1 ¼ cup almond flour

- ½ cup raw honey
- ½ cup coconut flour
- ½ cup applesauce
- 1/3 cup coconut oil
- ½ teaspoon baking powder
- ½ teaspoon sea salt

Cinnamon Frosting

- 3 tablespoons of raw honey
- 1 cup coconut oil
- Dash of sea salt
- 2 teaspoons cinnamon

Directions

1. Preheat oven to 350 °F. Place muffin cups in baking can. Mix all the ingredients in a mixing bowl. Beat on medium using a hand mixer until smooth then fill muffin cups to three fourth of its size with the mixture and bake for 30 minutes.

2. Take the cupcakes out and let it cool completely. Make the frosting by combining all the frosting ingredients in a mixing bowl and beat on medium speed using a hand mixer for 30 seconds.

3. Ice the cupcakes and serve.

Paleo Cheesecake With Blackberry Compote (244 Calories Per Serving)

Makes 10 Servings

Ingredients

For the Crust

- 2 tablespoons of raw honey
- 1 ½ cups raw almonds
- 10 medjool dates
- ½ teaspoon sea salt

Filling

- 2/3 cup raw honey
- ½ cup fresh squeezed lemon juice
- 3 cups cashews soaked
- ½ cup coconut oil, softened
- 1 tablespoon vanilla extract

Compote

- 1 teaspoon vanilla extract
- 3 cups blackberries
- 2 tablespoons raw honey
- 1/4 cup water

Directions

Making the Crust

1. Put almonds in a food processor and process for about 5 seconds. Add the honey and dates and blend until the dough sticks together. Take a pan and press the dough

into the pan and along the sides.

2. Use parchment paper in between the dough and fingers in order to avoid dough from sticking to hands. Keep the crust in the refrigerator. Start with the other layers.

Making the filling

1. Put cashews in a food processor and process for about 5 seconds.

2. Add the remaining filling ingredients and process until very smooth then empty the filling into the crust. Keep the top smooth and put it in the refrigerator.

Making the compote

1. Put blackberries and water in a medium sized saucepan and heat over medium heat. Let the berries cook for 20 minutes while stirring at regular intervals. Add the vanilla extract and raw honey and stir to mix.

2. Put the berry mixture in a mesh strainer. Put the strainer over a bowl. Apply pressure to the mixture with the back of a spoon and extract as much of the liquid as possible. Empty the berry compote over the top of the filling layer.

3. Be sure it is evenly distributed on the crust layer. Let it cool in the fridge for 2 hours then take it out and serve.

Paleo Dark & Salty Caramel Pots (327 Calories Per Serving)

Makes 2 Servings

Ingredients

Dark Chocolate Cake Pots

Few dashes of cinnamon

- 1 tablespoon coconut palm sugar
- 1 cup sifted fine blanched almond flour
- ½ teaspoon sea salt
- ½ teaspoon vanilla extract
- ½ cup canned coconut milk
- ½ teaspoon baking soda
- ¼ cup organic palm shortening
- 2 organic free-range eggs
- 1 cup dark chocolate chips

Directions

1. Preheat oven to 350 degrees. Mix almond flour, coconut palm sugar, cinnamon, baking soda and salt in a medium size bowl, stir together and put aside.

2. Mix chocolate chips and coconut milk in a separate bowl. Melt using the double boiler method and put aside. Stir in the organic palm shortening, vanilla and eggs into the melted chocolate mixture. Fold the dry ingredients into the melted chocolate mixture and stir until completely mixed. Put the batter into a piping bag, cut off the corner and squeeze the batter into the mason jars until they are about 2/3 full. Bake for 25 minutes.

3. Arrange the Paleo Dark and Salty Caramel Pots. Scrape an oversized dollop of Paleo Whipped Cream on top of the cake, Drizzle Paleo Caramel Sauce on top and serve.

Paleo Salted Caramel Sauce

Ingredients

- ½ teaspoon vanilla extract
- ½ cup canned coconut milk
- ½ cup grass-fed butter
- 1 cup coconut sugar

Directions

1. Mix coconut milk and butter in a pan over low heat. Once the butter has melted, add the vanilla extract, coconut sugar and salt; stir until mixed. Bring the mixture to a boil and boil for 3 minutes. Remove from the heat and stir until the mixture becomes smooth. The more the mixture cools, the more it thickens.

Paleo Whipped Cream

Ingredients

- *1 tablespoon light raw honey*
- *1 can coconut milk cream*
- 1 teaspoon vanilla extract

Directions

1. Put the can of coconut milk and the metal bowl in the refrigerator overnight. Invert the can upside down, open it, drain coconut water and spoon out the remaining cream into the chilled bowl. Add vanilla and honey. Take a hand mixer and beat together the ingredients in a medium speed. Stop when combined and creamy.

Conclusion

Thank you again for buying this book!

I hope this book was able to help you to understand what the paleo diet is all about and simple recipes that you can try at home as you begin your journey to living a paleo lifestyle.

Finally, if you enjoyed this book, please take the time to share your thoughts and post a review on Amazon. It'd be greatly appreciated!

Thank you and good luck!

Sarah

Bonus Gift For YOU

My **FREE** Gift to You! As a way of saying thank you for downloading my book I am willing to give you access to a selected group of readers who receive inspiring and life-changing kindle e-books for FREE. How would you feel being part of this group? How would it feel to be the first to know when I release fresh new content on health solutions, personal development and buisness strategies? How would it feel to get **instant access to this content for FREE**? It would feel great, wouldn't it? Of course it would.

You may ask yourself **WHY** I would give away books for **FREE** that I spent a lot of time and energy on writing. It's simple: **I want to spread the word**. AMAZON allows kindle authors to promote their newly released books by offering them to customers for free. Yet this is only allowed for a short period of time. Within this timeframe, we are able to spread the word quickly - and allowing users to download thousands and thousands of copies. When this promotion time is over, these books will revert to their normal selling price. That's exactly why you will **benefit from being the first to know** when they can be downloaded for FREE! So are you ready for your gift? You are just one click away from joining this elite group. I promise, it's for **FREE**. Follow the link below and simply enter your email address to start receiving really awesome content:

Click here to get instant access!

Thank you and enjoy!

Sarah

Made in the USA
Lexington, KY
07 July 2015